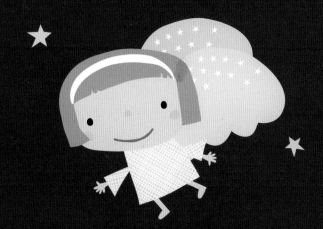

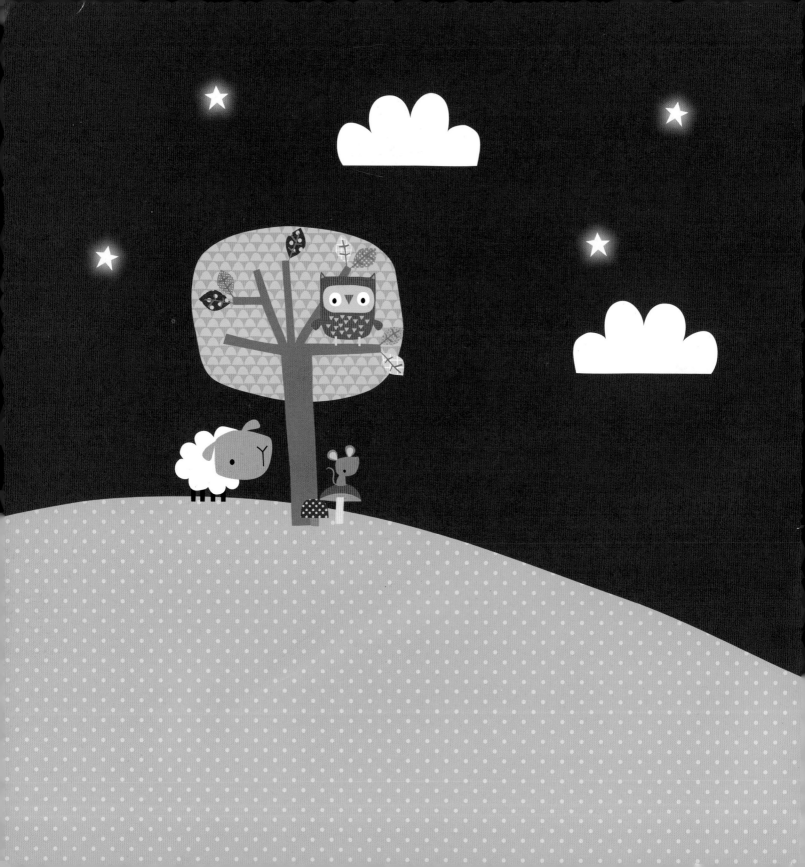

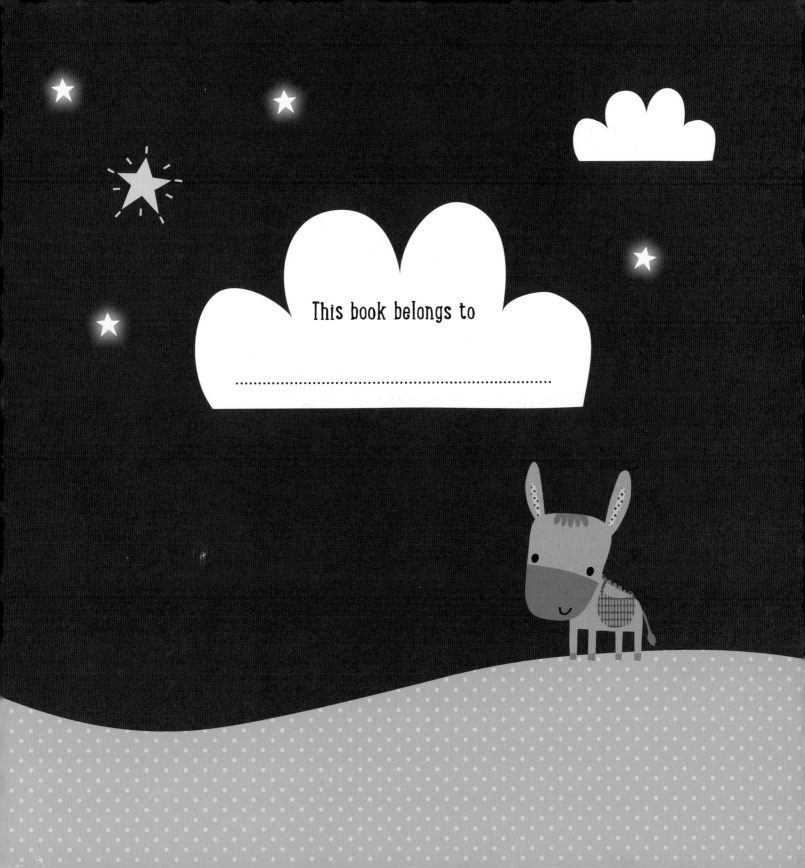

This book belongs to

....

THE STORY OF
CHRISTMAS

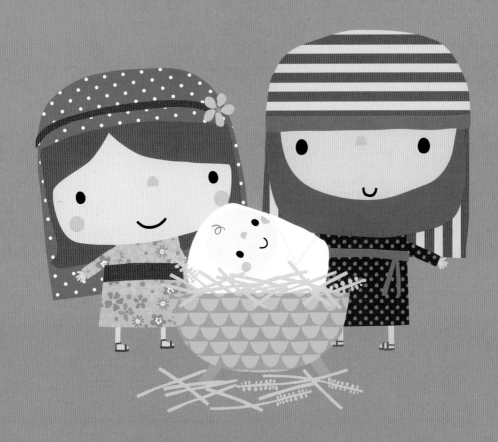

Dawn Machell • Hayley Down

make
believe
ideas

THE ANGEL'S NEWS

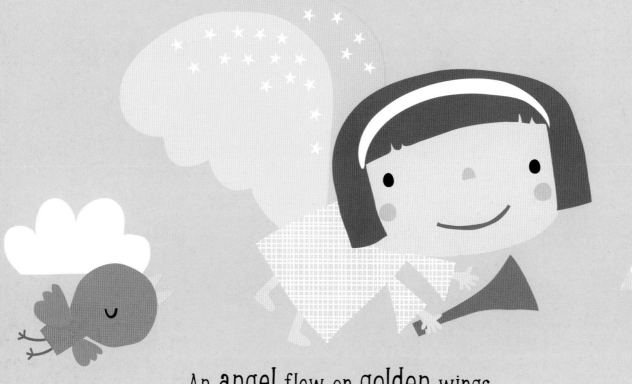

An **angel** flew on **golden** wings
to tell Mary **surprising** things:
"My dear, you are God's **chosen** one —
and you are **pregnant** with His Son."

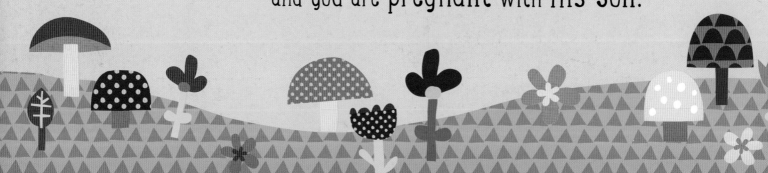

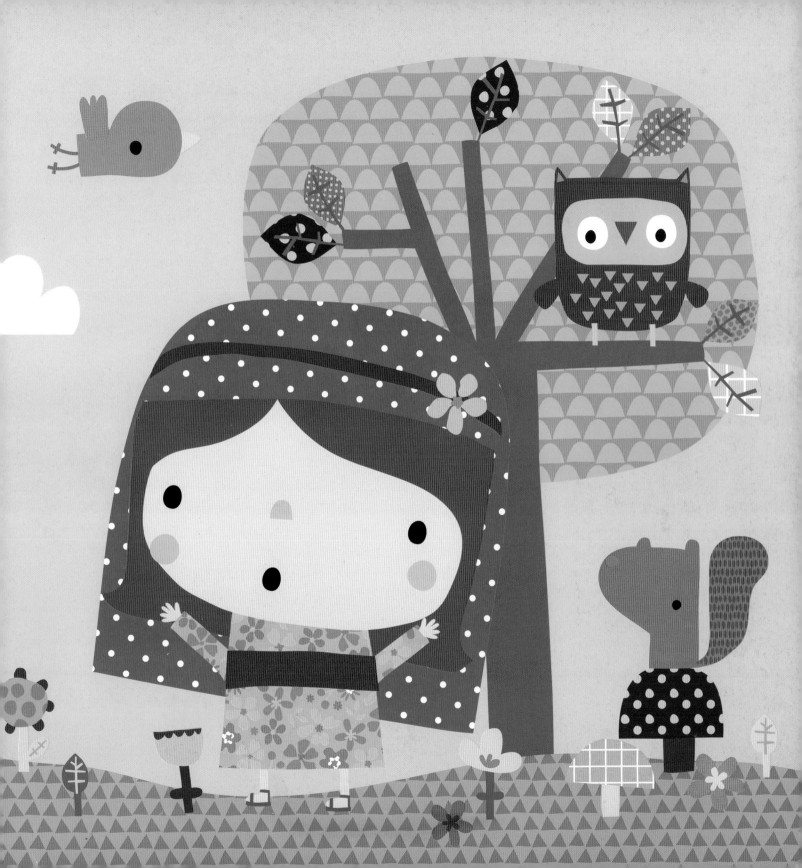

MARY AND ELIZABETH

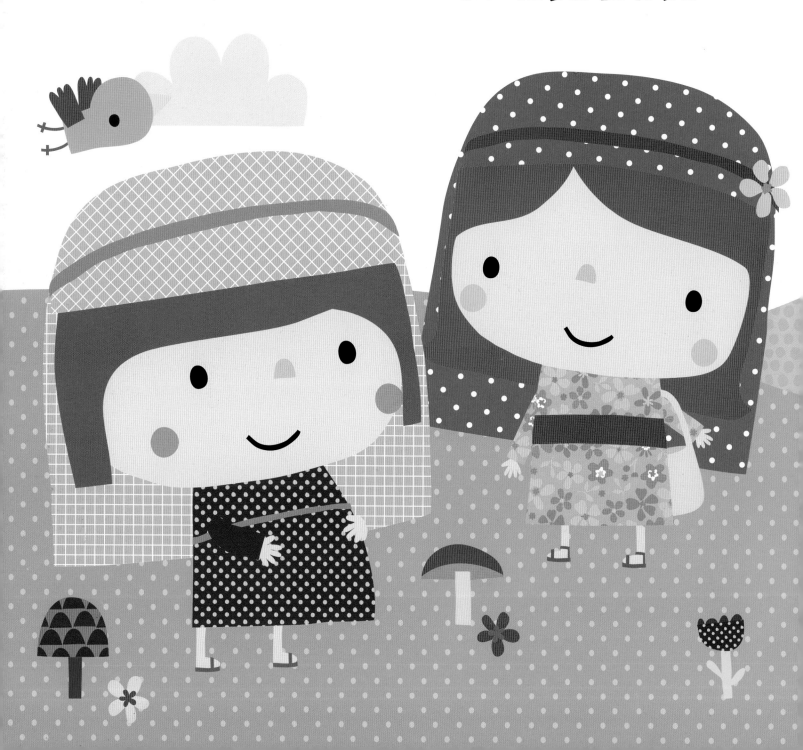

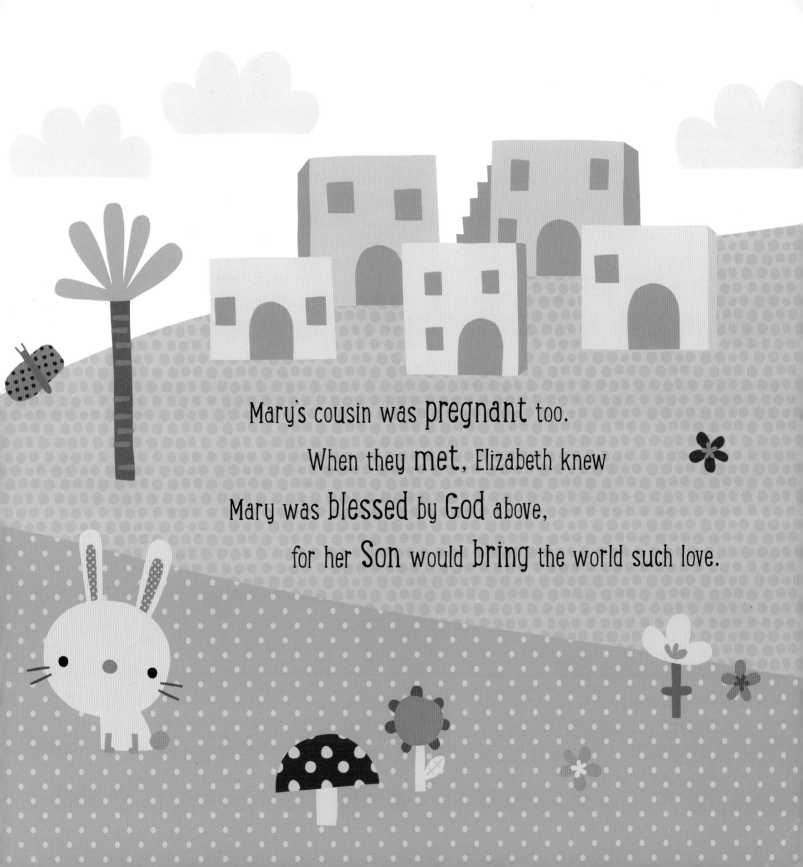

Mary's cousin was **pregnant** too.

When they **met**, Elizabeth knew

Mary was **blessed** by God above,

for her **Son** would **bring** the world such love.

JOURNEY TO BETHLEHEM

A new law meant Joseph must go

on a trip that was long and slow.

He took Mary to Bethlehem,

with a little donkey helping them.

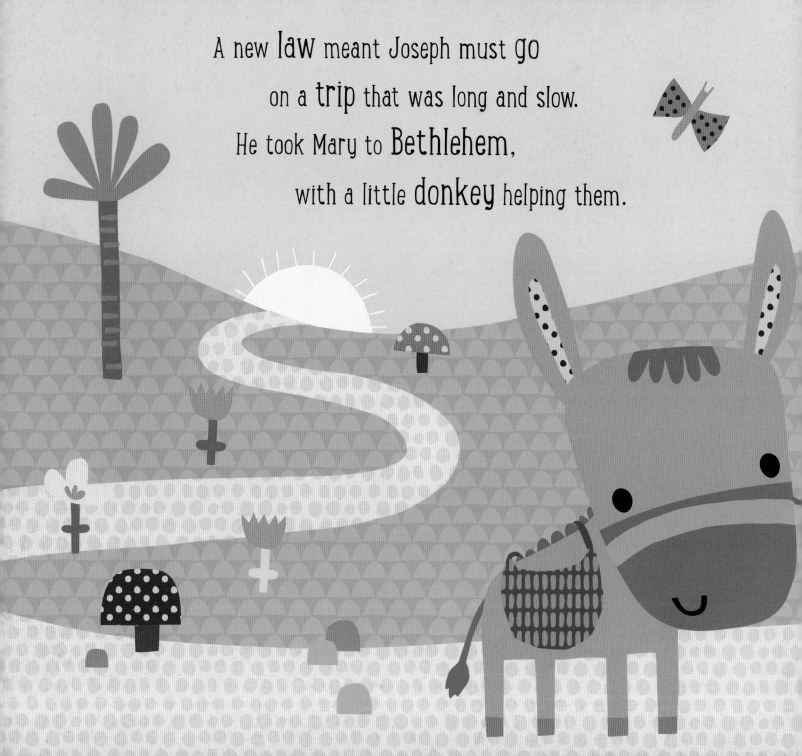

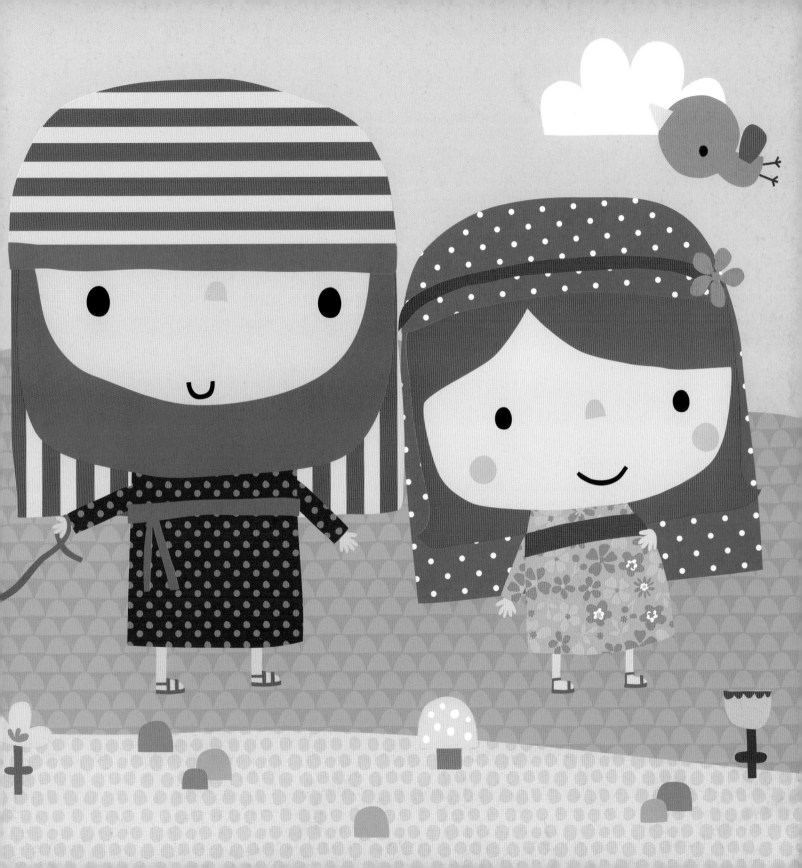

FINDING THE STABLE

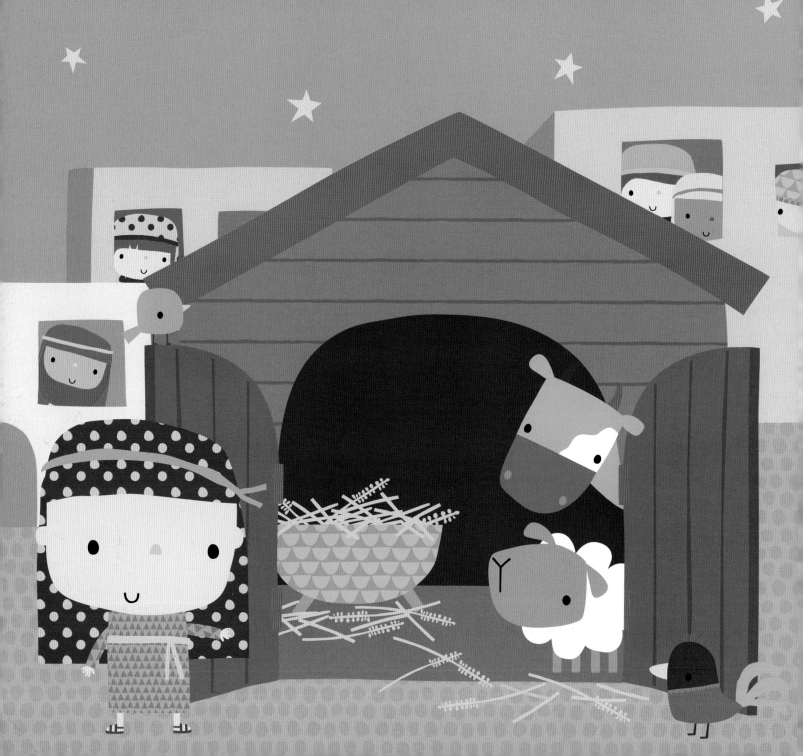

In Bethlehem no rooms were free
for Joseph and his family.
At last, they found a place to stay:
a warm, dry stable filled with hay.

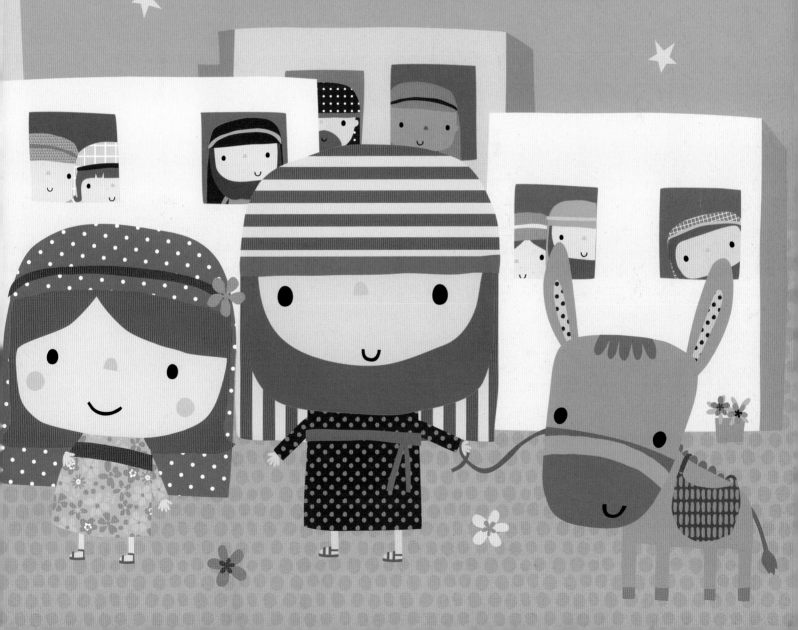

JESUS IS BORN!

Jesus was born that very night
under a **star** that shone so **bright**.
When it was time to **rest** His head,
they used a **manger** for His bed.

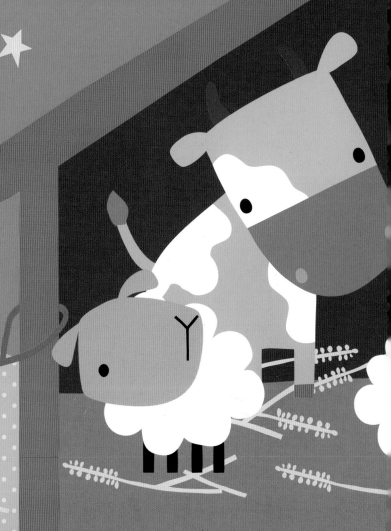

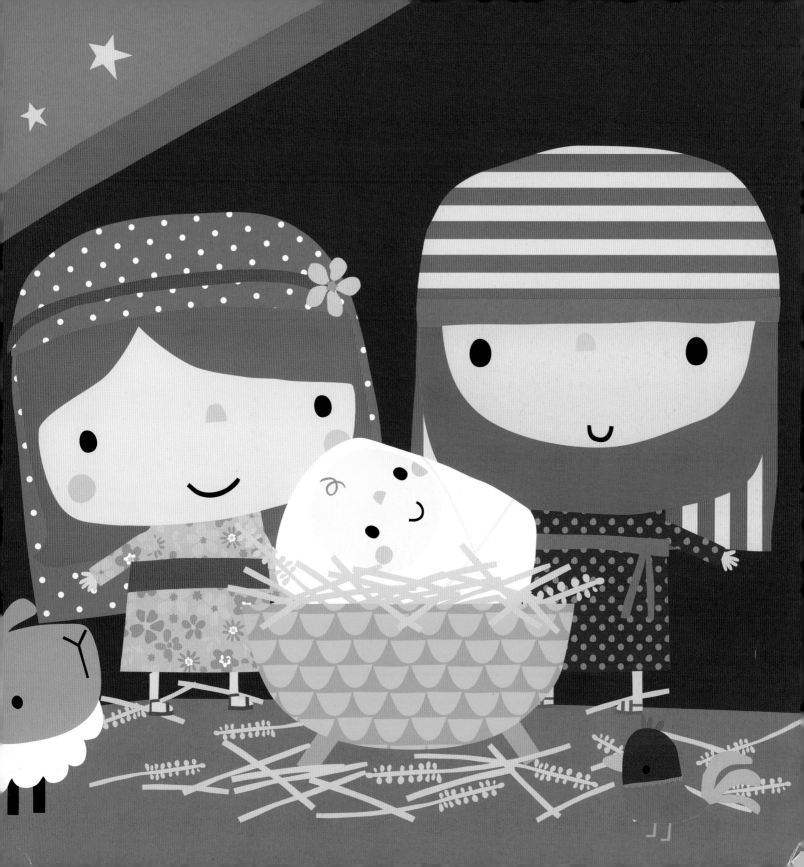

THE ANGELS' MESSAGE

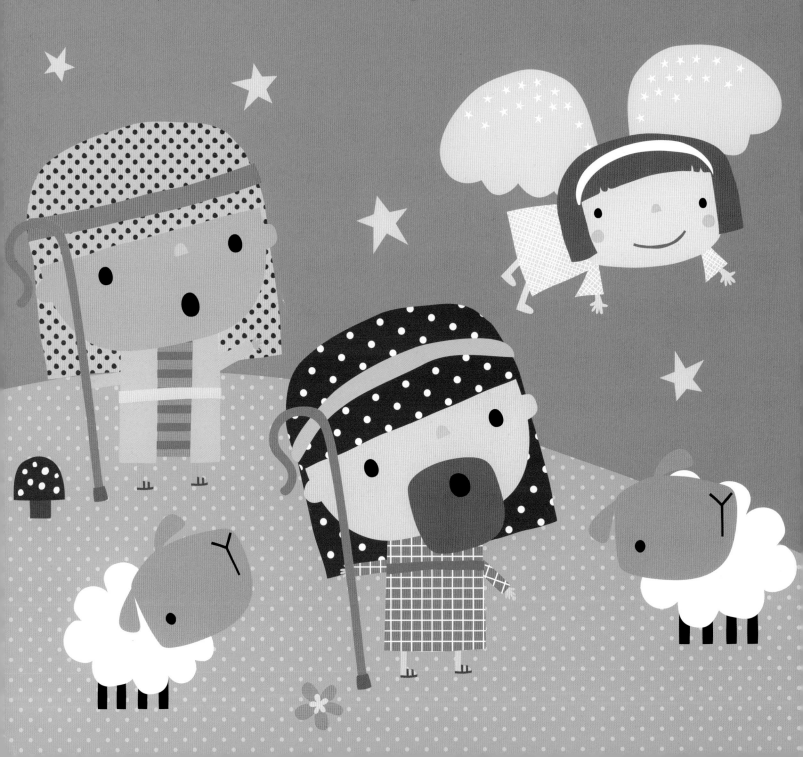

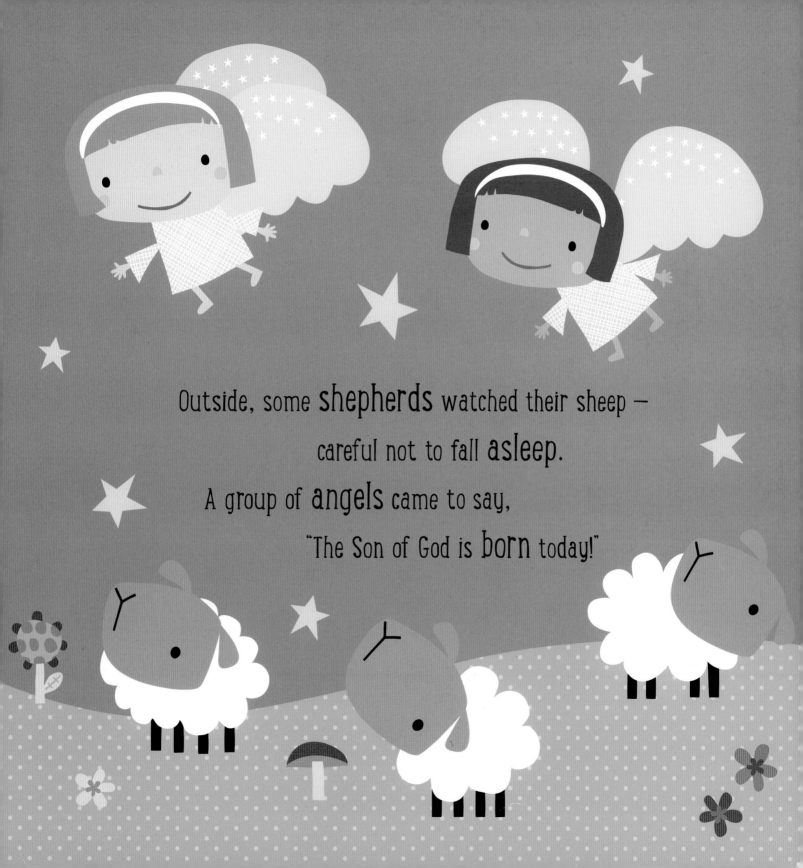

Outside, some **shepherds** watched their sheep —
careful not to fall **asleep**.
A group of **angels** came to say,
"The Son of God is **born** today!"

THE SHEPHERDS' VISIT

The shepherds rushed to see the boy,

who was to bring the world such joy.

They left and then told everyone

that they had met God's only Son.

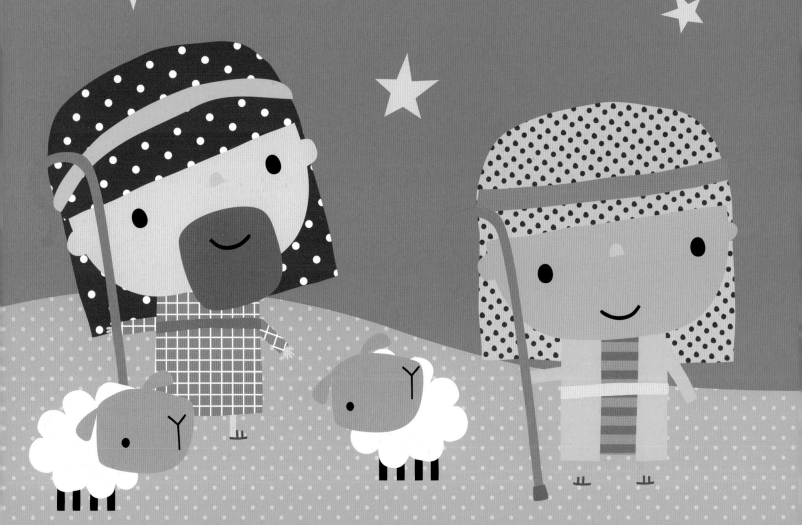

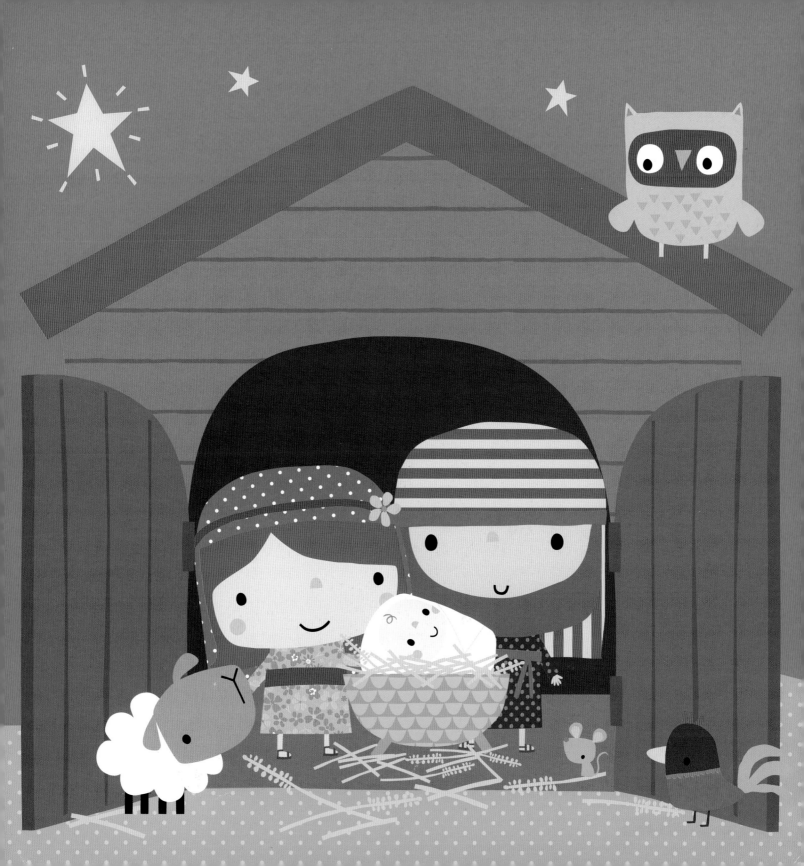

FOLLOWING THE STAR

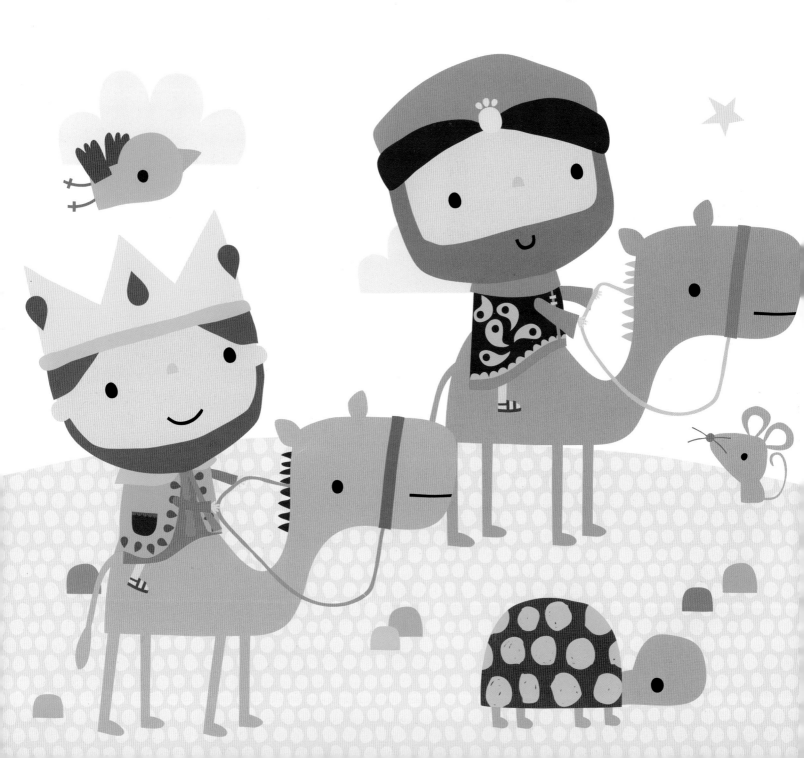

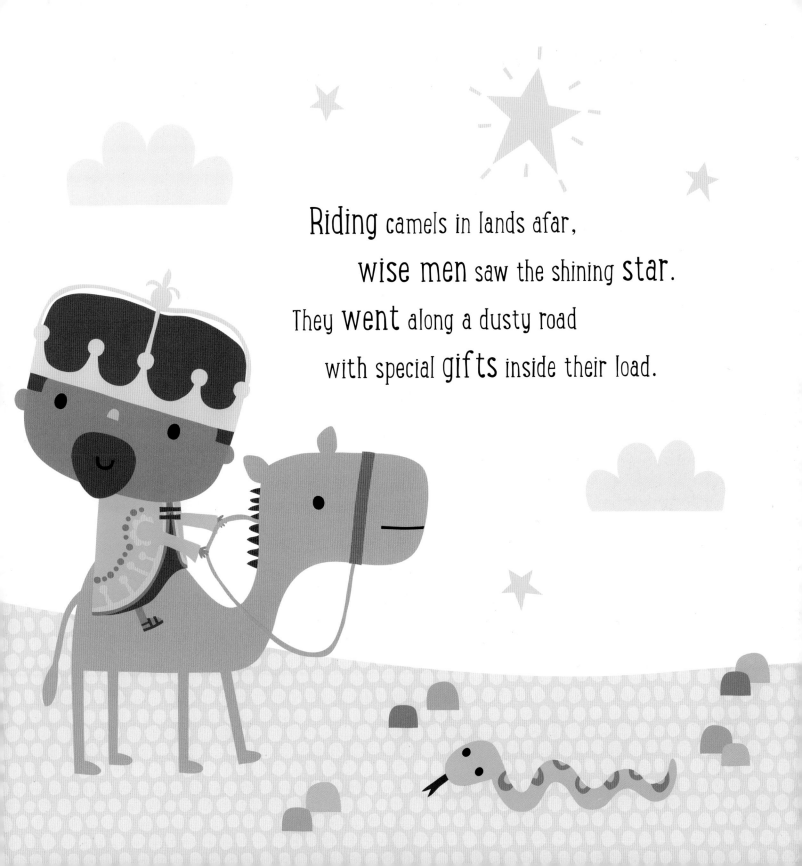

Riding camels in lands afar,
wise men saw the shining star.
They went along a dusty road
with special gifts inside their load.

GIVING GIFTS

They met the boy and bowed their heads.
Overjoyed, the wise men said,
"This is God's Son, as was foretold!
Please take this frankincense, myrhh, and gold."

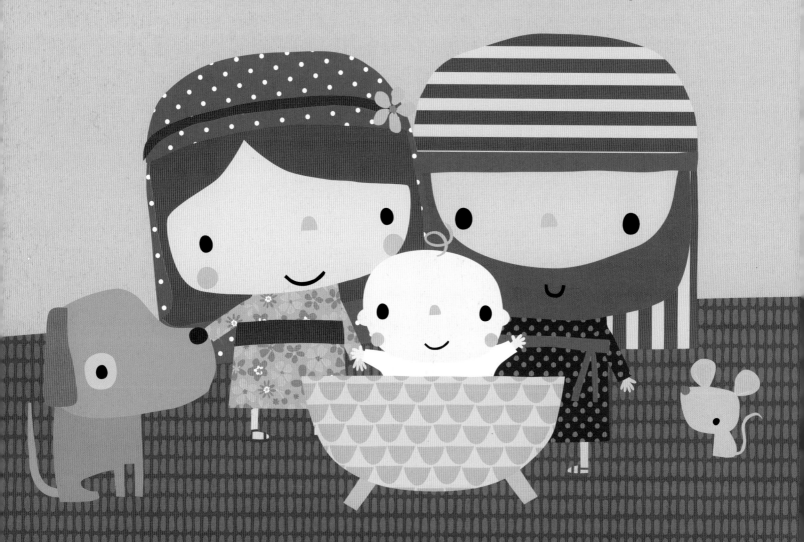

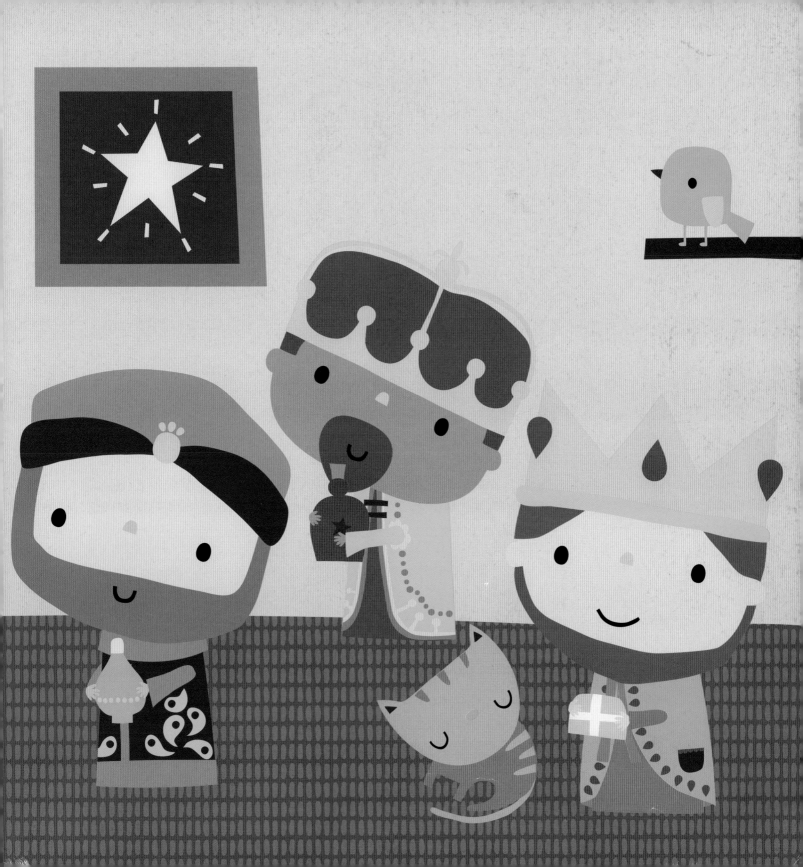

JESUS HAS RISEN!

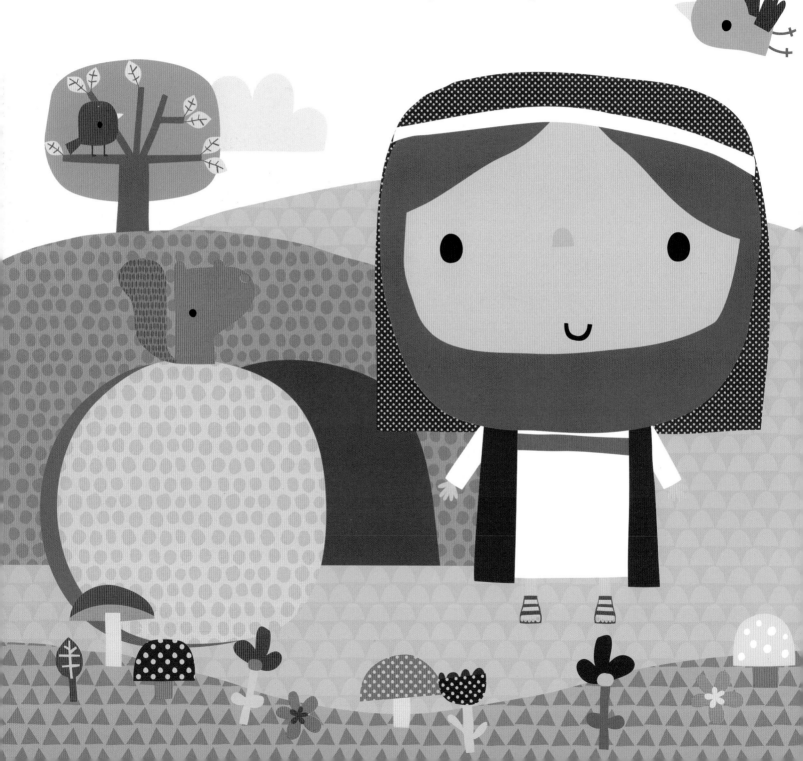

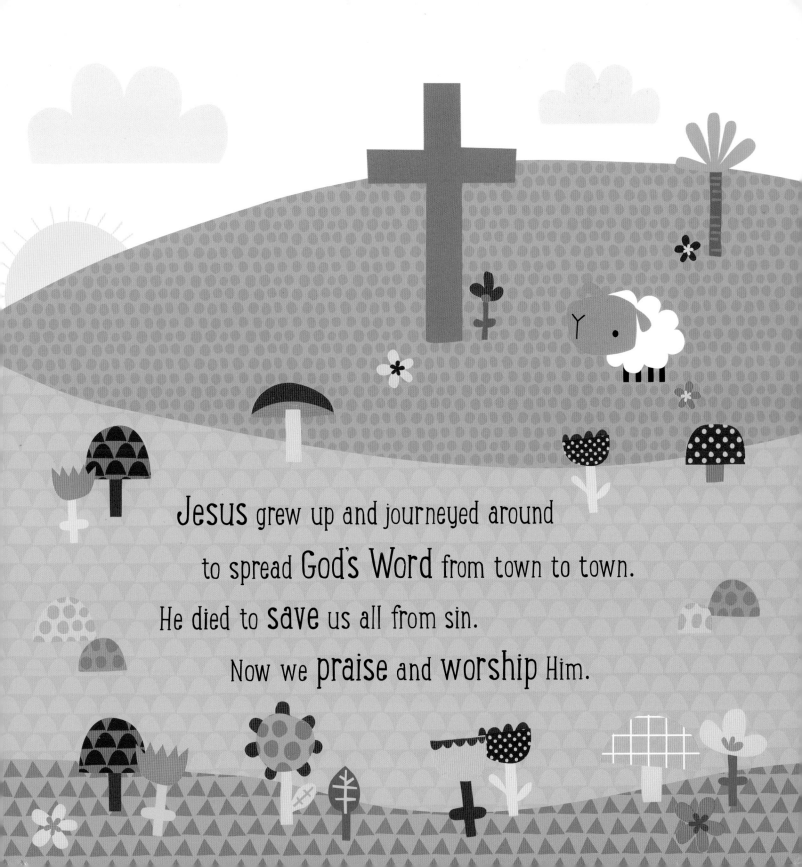

Jesus grew up and journeyed around
to spread God's Word from town to town.
He died to save us all from sin.
Now we praise and worship Him.

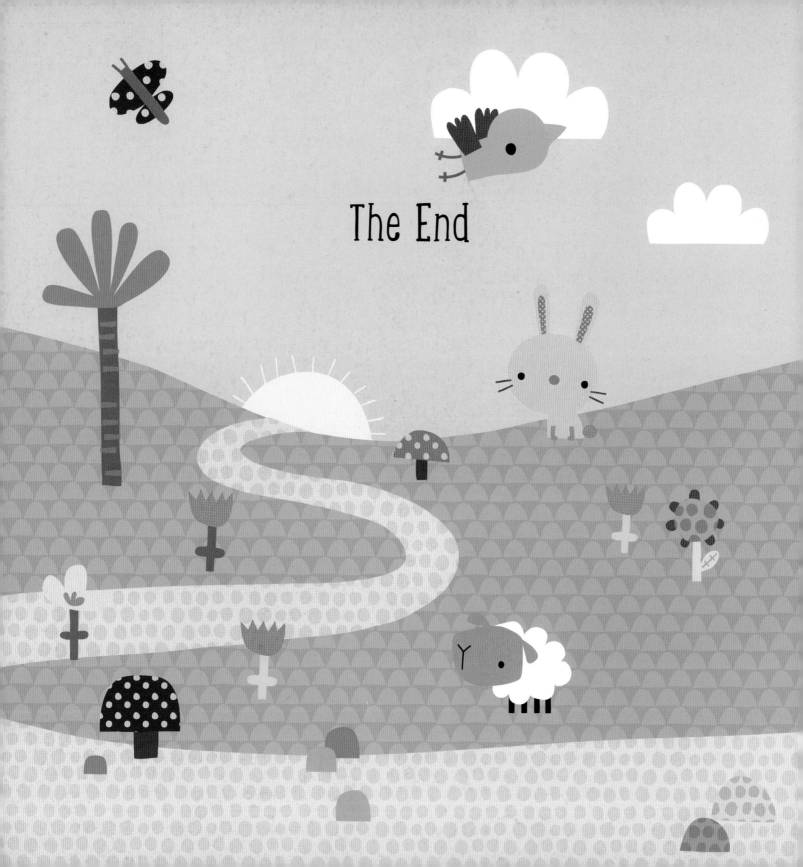

The End

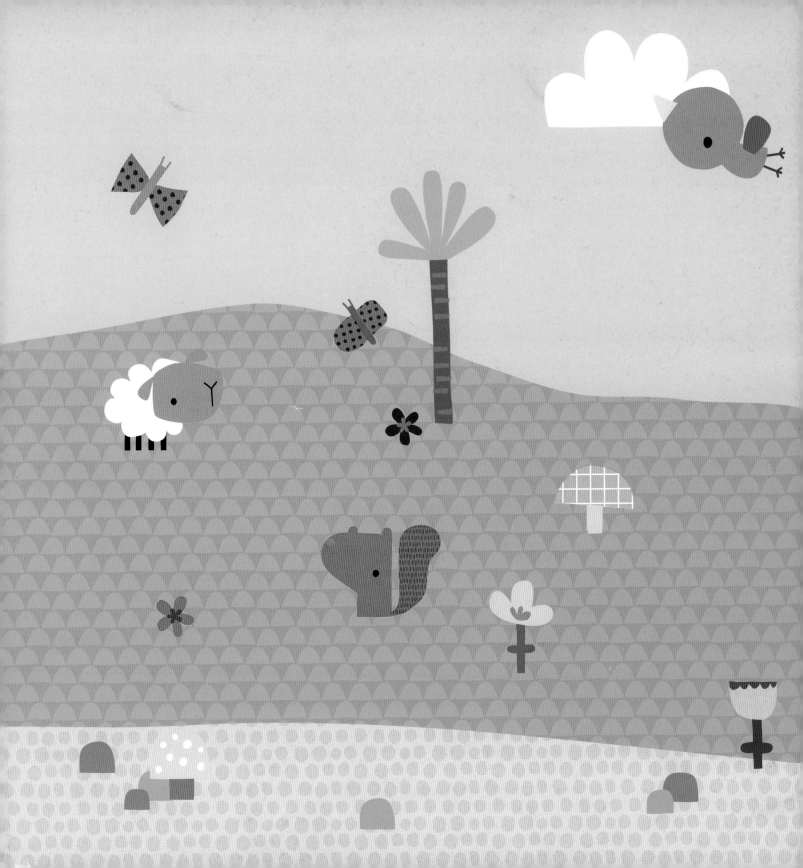

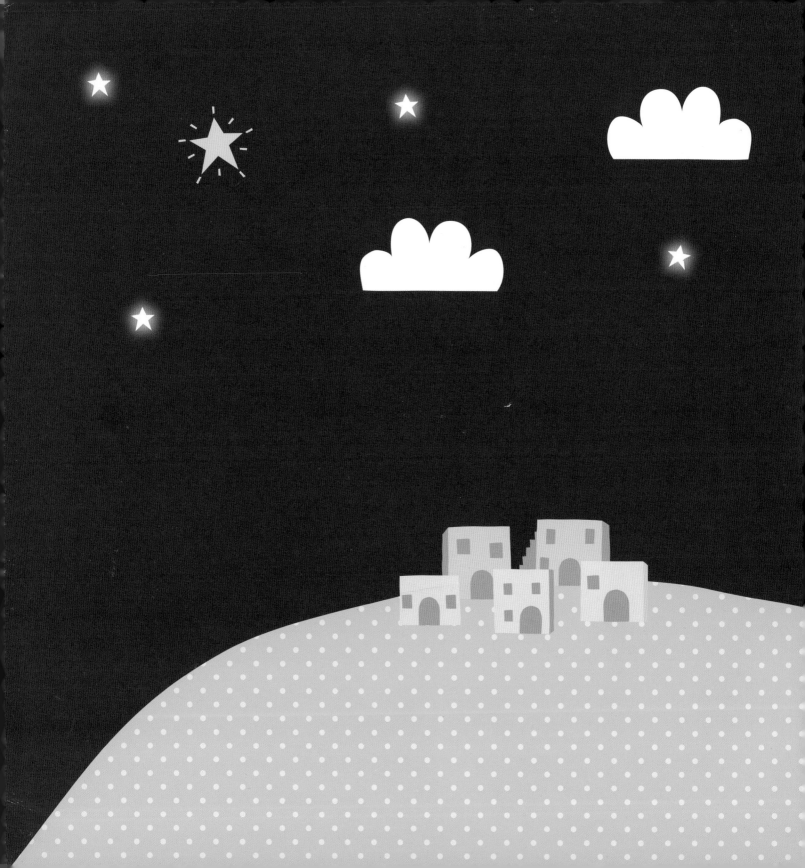

YOUNG PROFILES

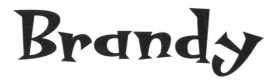

Lori Kinstad Pupeza
ABDO Publishing Company

visit us at
www.abdopub.com

Published by ABDO Publishing Company 4940 Viking Drive, Edina, Minnesota 55435.
Copyright © 1999 by Abdo Consulting Group, Inc. International copyrights reserved in
all countries. No part of this book may be reproduced in any form without written
permission from the publisher.

Printed in the United States.

Photo credits: AP/Wide World; Shooting Star

Edited by Paul Joseph
Contributing editor A.T. McKenna

Library of Congress Cataloging-in-Publication Data

Pupeza, Lori Kinstad
    Brandy / Lori Kinstad Pupeza
    p. cm. -- (Young profiles)
    Includes index.
    Summary: A biography of the award-winning young singer who is also the star
of the television series, "Moesha."
    ISBN 1-57765-323-8 (hardcover)
    ISBN 1-57765-335-1 (paperback)
    1. Brandy--Juvenile literature. 2. Singers--United States--Biography--Juvenile
literature. [1. Brandy. 2. Singers. 3. Actors and actresses. 4. Afro-Americans--
Biography.] I. Title. II. Series.
    ML3930.B77P87 2000
    782.42164'092--dc21
    [B]
                                           98-30894
                                               CIP
                                             MN AC

Contents

Brandy 4

Profile of a Young Star 6

Nominations and Awards 8

Growing Up 10

First Steps 12

A First Album 14

Honors and Awards 16

Role Models 18

Making It Big 20

Moesha 22

Cinderella 24

Never Say Never 26

Reaching for the Stars 28

Glossary 30

Fun Facts 31

Index 32

Brandy

Brandy R. Norwood is one of the hottest young stars today. She is one of very few people who have both a successful singing and acting career. She has two hit albums. She has a television program called *Moesha* that four million fans tune into each week. And she has received countless **nominations** and awards. She starred in the television movie *Cinderella*. Brandy started her own production company, along with the Norwood Kids Foundation, a nonprofit **organization** dedicated to serving young people.

Brandy has won the respect of many well-known people in the music, television, and film industry. Everything that she has a part in is an instant hit. The bubbly 19 year old has come a long way, but admits that she still has a lot to learn about handling fame and popularity. Brandy has learned a lot about being true to herself, and is thankful for everything she's been able to **accomplish**.

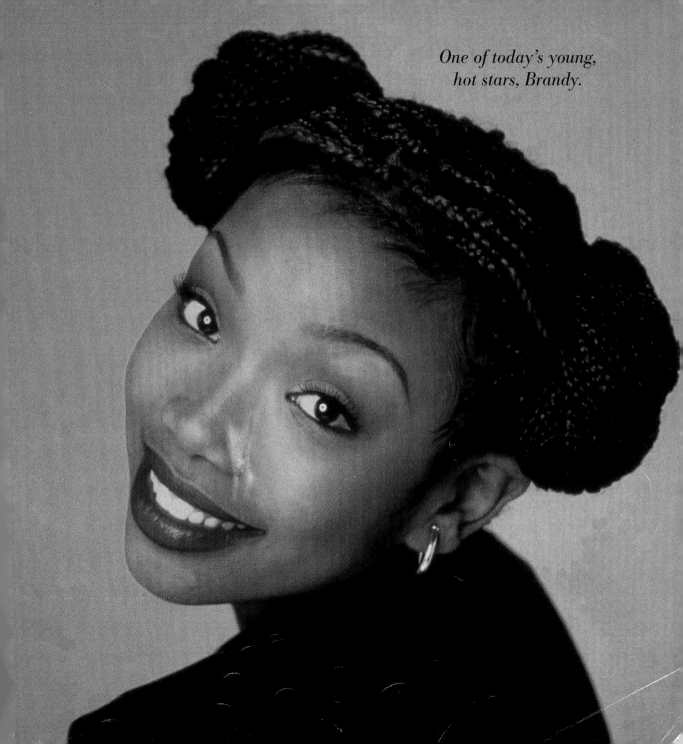

*One of today's young,
hot stars, Brandy.*

Profile of a
Young Star

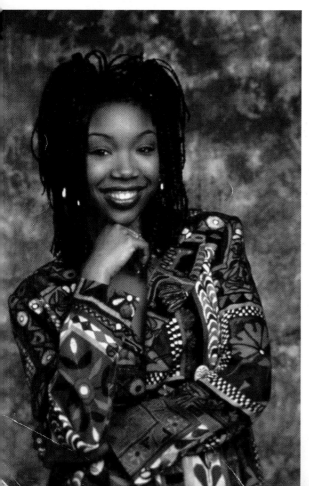

Brandy R. Norwood
Birth date: February 11, 1979
Birth Place: Macomb, Mississippi
Current Home: Los Angeles,
California
Education: Pepperdine University,
Malibu, California
Major: psychology and music
Family: mother Sonja, father Willie,
Sr., and brother Willie, Jr., also called
Ray J

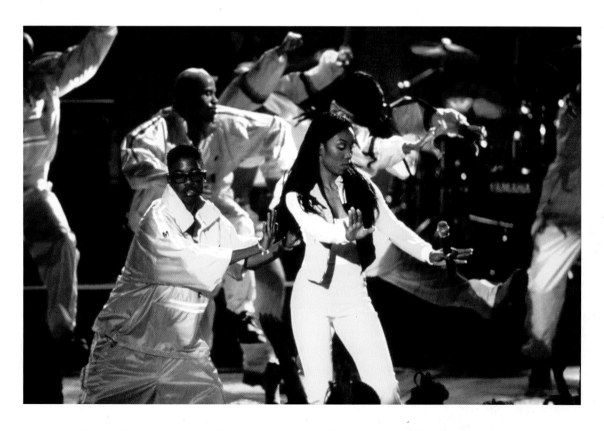

Brandy can do it all—act, sing, and perform. Here she is doing a performance at the Grammy Awards.

Nominations and Awards

Grammy Award Nominations
- Best New Artist
- Best R&B Performance

American Music Awards
- Favorite New Artist–Soul R&B

NAACP Image Awards
- Outstanding New Artist
  - 26th annual NAACP Image Awards Nominations
- TV: Outstanding Comedy: *Moesha*
- TV: Best Comedy Actress: Brandy (*Moesha*)

MTV Movie Awards
- Best Song ("Sittin' Up in My Room" from the *Waiting to Exhale* sound track)

Nickelodeon Award
- Favorite Singer

Soul Train Awards (first annual "Lady of Soul" awards)
- Best R&B/Single, Solo
- R&B/Soul Song of the Year for "I Wanna Be Down"
- Best R&B/Soul New Artist
- R&B/Soul Album of the Year, Solo
- Best New Artist of the Year

Soul Train Award (second annual "Lady of Soul" awards)
    Entertainer of the Year
Billboard Video Awards
    "I Wanna Be Down"
    "Baby"
Billboard Awards
    Best New Artist, R&B
    Best R&B Female
New York Children's Choice Award
    received from the young people of
        New York and New Jersey
MTV Video Music Awards
    Best Rap Video, "I Wanna Be Down"
        (featuring MC Lyte, Queen
        Latifah and Yo-Yo)
    Best Choreography, "Baby"

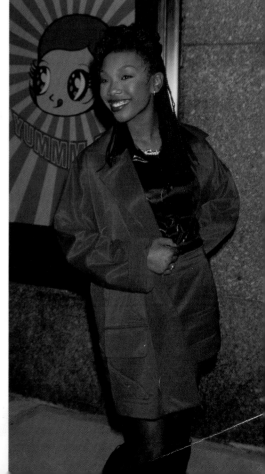

Brandy has received many awards and nominations in her short career.

Growing Up

Brandy was born in Macomb, Mississippi, but early in her life her family moved to Carson, California. Brandy has been singing since she was a child. Brandy's father is a minister, and she grew up singing in her father's church. Her father has a wonderful singing voice, which has been passed on to both Brandy and her brother Ray J. Brandy's mother, who is now her **manager**, said "Brandy grew up singing. She could sing before she could talk."

Brandy first knew that she wanted to become a singer when she saw Whitney Houston perform on TV. She turned to her father and said "Daddy, Daddy, I sing like her a little bit. I want to go out and be a singer like her." She also expressed interest in acting. Brandy's parents listened to her, and brought her to talent shows. Her parents have always been supportive of her dreams, and at age 11, Brandy was in her first movie. She appeared in the comedy *Arachnophobia*.

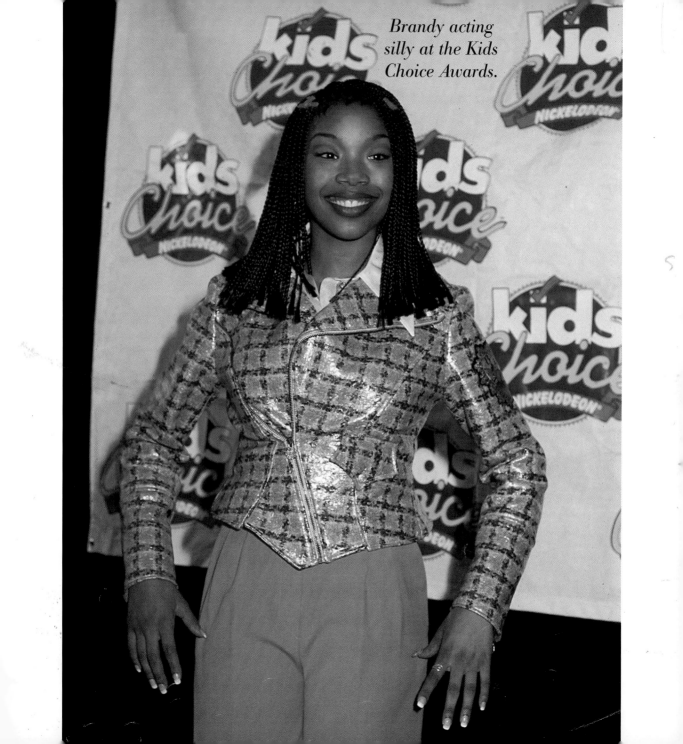

Brandy acting silly at the Kids Choice Awards.

First Steps

Brandy's rising stardom didn't happen overnight. She worked hard in order to make her talent known. Brandy said of her beginnings in the business, "I started going out and doing a lot of talent shows and stuff like that and eventually I ran into a producer. He started shopping me around in L.A. when I was 11 to different record companies and at the age of 14, I came to Atlantic Records and that's where I got my record deal."

Brandy would be working with one of the most **prestigious** record labels in the business. They saw her as the next huge success. Also in 1993 she got her first role in television. She played in the short-lived TV show *Thea*. The young talent was on her way to becoming a star. Brandy couldn't wait to get started on her first album called simply *Brandy*.

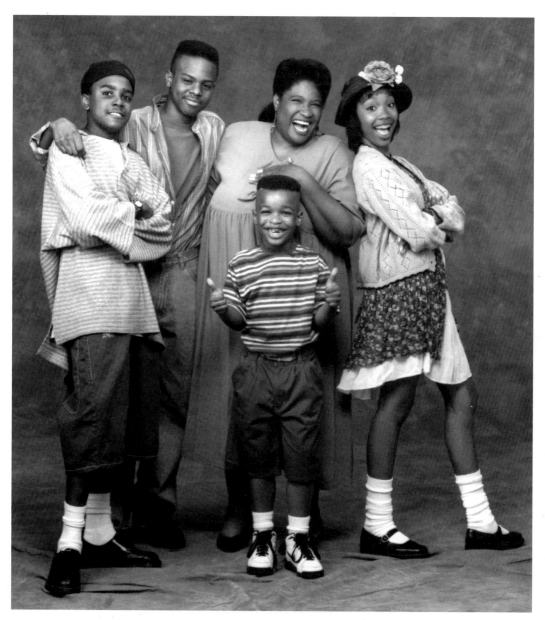

Brandy (far right) performed in the TV show Thea.

A First Album

The album *Brandy* sold over four million copies, and went platinum. It seemed like everybody loved her music. Her first single, "I Wanna Be Down," went gold. Another single, "Baby," came into the Billboard's pop charts at number 60. Not long after, it jumped to number five on the list.

Fans aren't the only ones to love her music. Critics and colleagues also think she has exceptional talent. Wayna Morris, of Boyz II Men, said of Brandy, "She's one of the baddest singers of the '90s. She's going to be out there for a long time."

Since recording her first album, Brandy has worked with huge stars like Michael Jackson, Lenny Kravitz, and Gladys Knight. Brandy also sang on the sound tracks for the movies *Waiting to Exhale* and *Batman Forever*.

*Opposite page: Brandy's first
album was a mega-hit.*

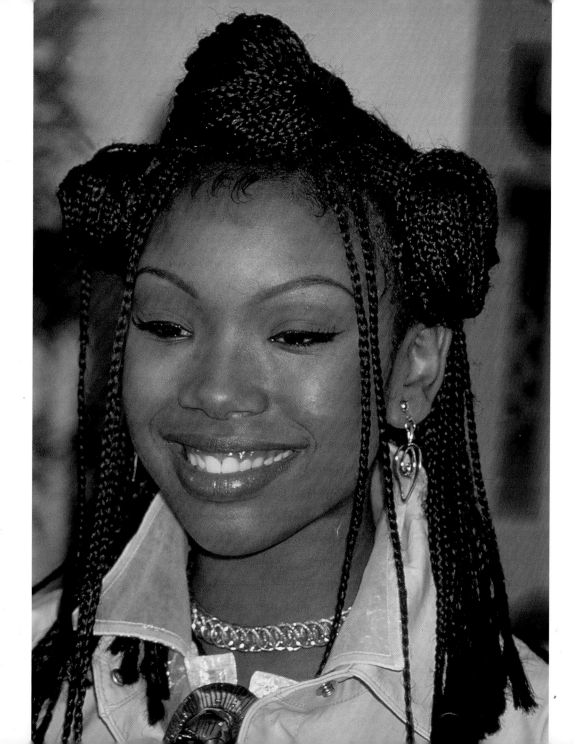

Honors and Awards

Brandy has won many awards for her talents. She was **nominated** for Grammy Awards, and won several NAACP Image Awards. She also has several Soul Train Awards, MTV Awards, and Billboard Awards. She's very proud of these honors, but feels that they aren't what is most important.

Being on top of the charts isn't what makes Brandy work hard. "If I can't feel it, then I won't sing it. And many of the songs heard were not me. They didn't express what I wanted to say at this point in my career [after *Brandy*]."

Brandy wants to feel a connection to her music, and her fans love her for it. She has six consecutive Top 10 singles, including two platinum hits, "Baby" and "Sittin' Up in My Room," and two gold hits, "I Wanna Be Down" and "Brokenhearted."

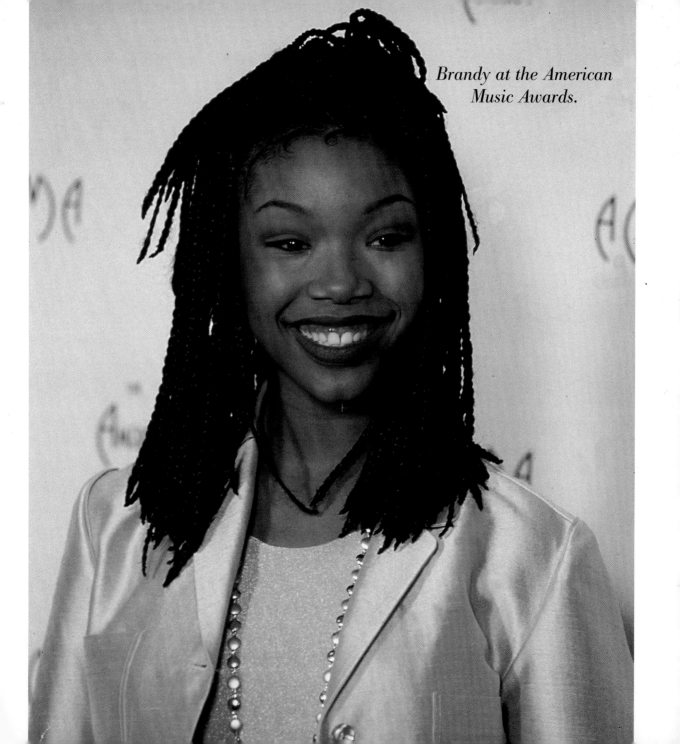

Brandy at the American Music Awards.

Role Models

All those awards came from a lot of hard work and **inspiration** from some of the best talents in show business. Brandy's biggest role model is Whitney Houston. She once said of Whitney in an interview that "I met her and cried. I'd been dying to meet her since I was a kid. . . . She is the beginning and ending of a singer. You can feel what she's saying. I try to perform exactly like her when I'm onstage."

Brandy has become a role model herself. She says that she never smokes cigarettes or drinks alcohol. She earns good grades and goes to church with her family when she's in town.

"I'm safe," she says. "Sometimes too safe. I want every move I make to be right. Like, I thought it was a good idea for me to go to the prom with Kobe Bryant (the Los Angeles Lakers All-Star guard). He's a good guy with a good image; comes from a good family. Every move that I make in my career, I want to make sure it complements me. That's why nothing really negative has come out of my life, because I try to make everything as right as I possibly can."

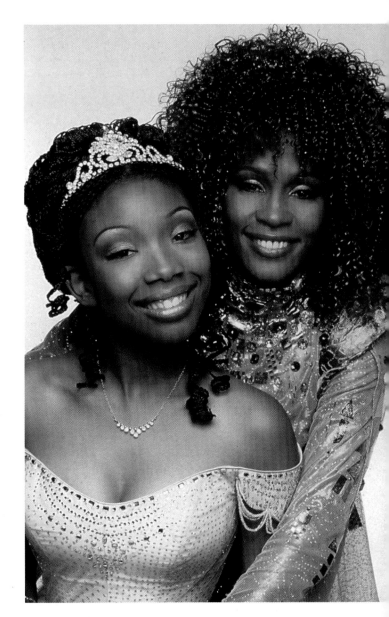

Brandy with her role model Whitney Houston when they worked together in Cinderella.

Making It Big

Fellow entertainers aren't Brandy's only role models. Her parents have played a large role in her life. Parents Willie and Sonja Norwood have become skilled **managers** of Brandy's career. They want her public image to reflect the smart, confident young woman who Brandy is in real life. "No one," Sonja said of her daughter, "no one is going to have the opportunity of taking the **principles** that we've instilled in my child and shape her into somebody else."

Through all of the Hollywood hype and shining lights, Brandy tries to make time for having fun. She loves being able to meet her heroes, like Whitney Houston, Celine Dion, and Mase. At a surprise party for her sixteenth birthday, she was showered with gifts from the members of Boyz II Men. She realizes how lucky she is, and her success still seems to shock her. "Most teens don't get this opportunity. This is, like, such a dream for me—I been dreamin' it since I was a young, young girl. Sometimes I wish somebody would pinch me."

Brandy with one of her heroes, Celine Dion.

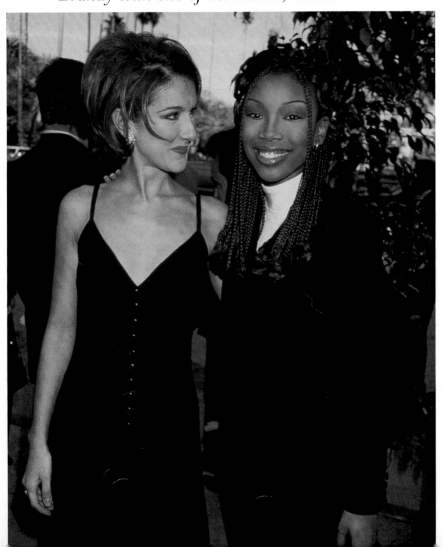

Moesha

Brandy has proven that she can not only make great music, but she can also act on an award winning television show. The TV show *Moesha* is the number one rated program on the UPN network. The sitcom is about the struggles that teenagers go through at home and school.

Brandy plays the leading role, Moesha Mitchell. Moesha is a teenage girl who lives in Los Angeles, California, with her father Frank, his new wife Dee, and her younger brother Myles. Moesha is adjusting to the new woman in their family, and developing a close relationship with her.

Moesha also hangs out with her best friend Kim and other friends at school, sometimes getting into trouble. The show *Moesha* takes a comic look at growing up in a modern world, through the eyes of a young woman.

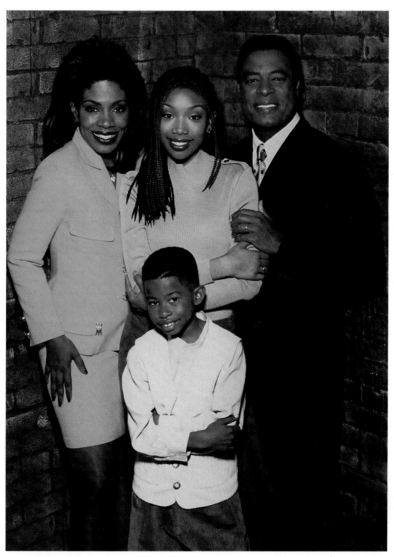

The cast from Moesha: on the left is Dee, played by Sheryl Lee Ralph; in the front is Myles, played by Marcus T. Paulk; in the middle is Moesha, played by Brandy; and on the right is Frank, played by William Allen Young.

Cinderella

In 1997, Brandy expanded her acting career by playing the lead role in the made for television movie, *Cinderella*. It was watched by more than 60 million people. ABC-TV said it was its biggest number one ratings win in over 10 years. The home video sold over one million copies. Brandy was the first African American to play the character of Cinderella.

Brandy was excited about acting in the movie. When she began working on the set, she felt she had to prove herself to the others there. "I don't think the producers really believed in me on *Cinderella*. I thought maybe they cast me because of my name or Whitney Houston wanted me in the part. I felt like I had to prove myself. There were dance rehearsals and music rehearsals, but on top of all that, I rehearsed every day, an hour on every song. And you know what? By the time we got to the studio to record the score, they were shocked. I wasn't just the girl Whitney hand-picked. I was a real singer."

Brandy gained much respect from the film and music **industries** with her acting and singing in *Cinderella*.

The cast from Cinderella.

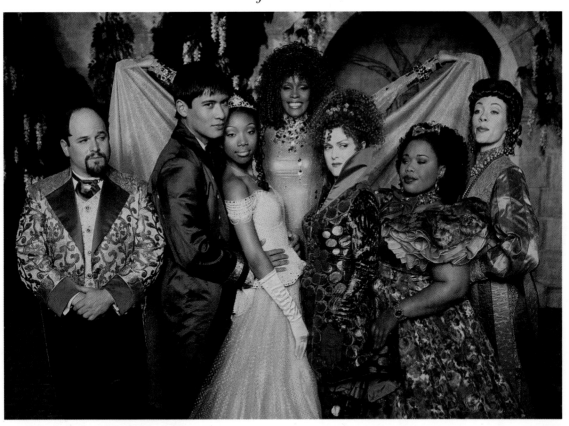

Never Say Never

Brandy continues to work on her singing career while acting on TV programs and movies. In 1998, she had a major role in the movie *I Still Know What You Did Last Summer*. Brandy also released her newest album at that time, called *Never Say Never*. She has grown both **physically** and **emotionally** since her first album Brandy.

"I'm not the little girl I was when I made my first record. My voice is a stronger instrument now, my vocals come from both my heart and **diaphragm**. My heart, because I've matured in the four years since the last album, I'm more emotionally there. The diaphragm because I've been practicing, doing more with my father, just strengthening my sound."

Brandy's new album is about a young woman trying to figure out life. Her stylish, funky lyrics echo her strong, melodic vocals. In the song "Top of the World," featuring hiphop star Mase, Brandy sings out with a slamming beat "Just tryin' to be me, doin' what I gotta do . . ."

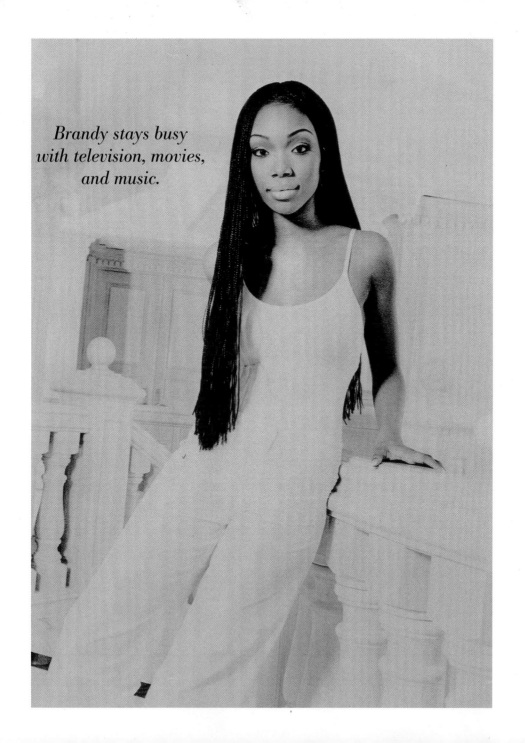

Brandy stays busy with television, movies, and music.

Reaching for the Stars

Even though Brandy is always busy singing and acting on television and in movies, she always remains true to herself. She only sings the kind of music that she loves, and acts in roles that she likes. Working in the entertainment business isn't always easy, and Brandy has had to deal with harsh critics and demanding roles. But because of all her hard work, she has accomplished many of her dreams.

Brandy says of it all, "I'm not going to lower my standards, I'll continue to surround myself with beautiful, positive people. It's hard being 19 sometimes in this business, because I'm more of an adult than a teenager; I have to stay focused. But I'm not boastful. I'm going to stay low, keep moving, and believe in God. As long as people can relate to my music, to

what I'm saying,
and feel the
groove, then I'll
know it was all
worth it."

*Brandy with her
mother.*

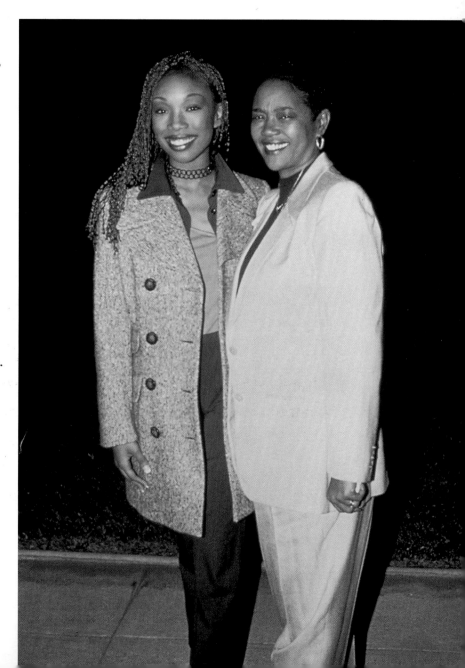

Glossary

Accomplish: to achieve or finish something.

Diaphragm: a muscle in the abdomen that helps a singer to sing loud.

Emotionally: having to do with feelings.

Established: started, or the beginning of something.

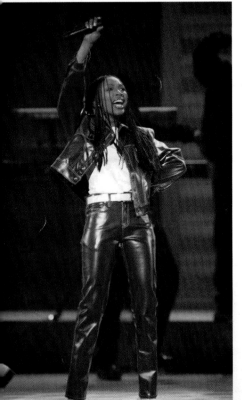

Brandy in concert.

Industries: types of businesses.

Inspiration: someone who has influenced someone else in a good way.

Manager: someone who manages, or takes care of someone else.

Nominations: chosen to be in the running for an award; being nominated is an honor in and of itself.

Organization: a business or club.

Physically: in a physical way.

Prestigious: having fame or dignity.

Principles: beliefs or codes that one has for oneself.

Fun Facts

Favorite artists: Whitney Houston, Mase (He's on Brandy's new album), Monica (She's also on her new album), Puffy, TLC, Boyz II Men, Mariah Carey, Fugees, Celine Dion, Alanis Morissette
Favorite movie: *The Bodyguard* with Whitney Houston
Favorite TV-shows: *Home Improvement, Family Matters*
First date: Kobe Bryant; prom night.

Visit Brandy on her official website:

www.atlantic-records.com

This is a must see website for all Brandy fans. Listen to her hit songs, get on her mailing list, join her fan club, checkout the fun chat-room! You may even get to chat with Brandy!

Pass It On

Tell readers around the country information you've learned about your favorite superstars. Share your little-known facts and interesting stories.
We want to hear from you!
To get posted on the ABDO Publishing Company Web site, E-mail us at "Adventure@abdopub.com"
Download a free screen saver at www.abdopub.com

Index

A

ABC-TV 24
Arachnophobia 10
Atlantic Records 12

B

"Baby" 9, 14, 16
Batman Forever 14
Billboard Awards
  9, 14, 16
Boyz II Men 20, 30
Bryant, Kobe 18, 30

C

Carson, California 10
church 10, 18
Cinderella 4, 24, 19, 25
critics 28

D

diaphragm 26
Dion, Celine 20, 30

F

family 10, 18, 19
fans 4, 16
film 4, 25

G

Grammy Awards 8, 16

H

Houston, Whitney 10,
  18, 20, 24, 30

I

*I Still Know What You Did
  Last Summer* 26
"I Wanna Be Down" 8, 9,
  14, 16

J

Jackson, Michael 14, 30

L

Los Angeles, California 6

M

Macomb, Mississippi 6,
  10
manager 10, 20
Moesha 4, 8, 22, 26
MTV 8, 9, 16

N

NAACP 8, 16
Nickelodeon 8
Norwood Kids Foundation
  4

P

parents 10, 20
producer 12, 24
production 4
public image 20

R

ratings 24
record companies 12
rehearsals 24
role model 18, 19, 20

S

school 22
Soul Train Awards 8, 16

T

talent shows 10, 12
television 4, 22, 24, 28
Thea 12, 13

U

UPN network 22

W

Waiting to Exhale 8, 14